Pain as a Means of Grace

Pain as a Means of Grace

MORRIS A. INCH

WIPF & STOCK · Eugene, Oregon

PAIN AS A MEANS OF GRACE

Copyright © 2009 Morris A. Inch. All rights reserved. Except for brief quotations in critical publications or reviews, no part of this book may be reproduced in any manner without prior written permission from the publisher. Write: Permissions, Wipf and Stock, 199 W. 8th Ave., Suite 3, Eugene, OR 97401.

Wipf and Stock Publishers
199 W. 8th Ave., Suite 3
Eugene, OR 97401

www.wipfandstock.com

ISBN 13: 978-1-60608-527-1

Manufactured in the U.S.A.

Contents

Preface / vii

Acknowledgment / ix

1. Paradise Lost / 1
2. The Sage / 14
3. The Passion Legacy / 25
4. Voices of the Martyrs / 37
5. A Reasoned Faith / 49
6. Highlights / 62

Bibliography / 71

Preface

Aristotle succinctly observed, "To perceive is to suffer" (De Anima). Consequently, we must come to grips with pain if we are to negotiate life meaningfully. In this regard, Paul encourages us: "But we know that in all things God works for the good of those who love him, who have been called according to his purpose" (Rom 8:28). It goes without saying that not all things are desirable in and of themselves. Conversely, they may serve as a means of realizing God's rich blessing.

We will explore this illusive subject first by way of paradise lost, since this serves to explain life as we encounter it. In other words, it provides a much needed reality check. After that, we turn to the classic narrative concerning the patriarch Job. In this connection, to account for why the godly suffer.

The passion narrative next invites our attention. As a result, we consider how suffering furthers God's redemptive purpose. The voices of the martyrs appear as a logical extension. In particular, we recall the martyrs' stalwart faith and confident witness. We then explore in more systematic fashion the apologetic concerns associated with suffering. Finally, we will review some of the highlights.

Since it is said that a story is the shortest way to truth, I will conclude these introductory remarks with a pertinent incident. A certain young couple was delighted that they would soon become parents. However, they were subsequently alerted to the fact that the child would be severely handicapped. They were understandably crestfallen.

The husband, who came across as a nominal Christian, summarily gave up on the idea of God's existence. His wife struggled with a troubled faith. They could not bring themselves to abort the fetus.

The baby was delivered. Time passed, and the parents came to appreciatively refer to the addition as their love child. This reflected not only their deep affection for the infant, but an enhanced relationship between them. In a manner of speaking, they had embraced pain as a means of grace.

We are thus primed for the discussion to follow. Initially, as noted above, with reference to paradise lost. In this connection, we should bear in mind that even small variations in initial conditions are calculated to have a disproportionately significant impact on subsequent events. Then, too, the fall was of tragic proportions.

Acknowledgment

I am again indebted to my beloved wife Joan, who has served as copy editor and proof reader.

1

Paradise Lost

I AM reminded of a youngster who habitually tuned in late to a conversation. As a result he had difficulty getting his bearings. It helps immeasurably to start from the beginning; in this instance, with paradise lost—so as to engage the topic of suffering.

Initially, consider *pain* as such. We first encounter it in conjunction with the Almighty's foreboding announcement to Eve: "I will greatly increase your pains in childbearing; with pain you will give birth to children. Your desire will be for your husband, and he will rule over you" (Gen 3:16). Physical pain is thus identified with *travail*. I have heard it said that a severe attack of kidney stones is the closest approximation for a male.

Then, too, pain is associated with emotional duress. In particular, to love and cherish becomes to desire and dominate. In other connections as well, so that the psalmist feels utterly forsaken; coupled, it would seem, with a sense of abject futility (cf. 22:1). Or, as otherwise expressed, he was in the depths of depression.

"What do you read?" the learned rabbi inquired in a manner characteristic of traditional inquiry.

"In the beginning God created the heaven and the earth," his student dutifully replied (Gen 1:1). *In the beginning* likely corresponds to *the time of the gods* in pagan literature. This was before humans made their appearance, and the gods characteristically jostled with one another for position. In this instance, God existed in solitary splendor. Moreover, he was lacking in nothing.

Qualifications aside, the Genesis account resembles other high god narratives. The term *high* god pertains to the supreme god in polytheistic religion, as well as the sole deity in monotheism. Additionally, the prime creation metaphor in the high god narratives is that of a potter casting his clay and fashioning a vessel.

I remember the scene well. We were looking on as a Hebron potter cast an amorphous lump of clay, paused momentarily in anticipation of what would transpire, and began to spin his wheel. Incidentally, he was referred to as *the old man*, considered a compliment in a society where age is revered. In astonishing fashion, a vessel soon began to take shape. Those observing murmured their approval

"What else do you read?" the mentor again inquired.

"Now the earth was formless and empty, darkness was over the surface of the deep," the youth responded, "and the Spirit of God was hovering over the waters" (v. 2). This combination of terms (*formless and empty*) is found only here and in Jeremiah 4:23, the former concerning the physical conditions and the latter of the disintegration of society resulting from the Babylonian invasion. In terms of analogy, it resembles the previously mentioned lump of clay.

Whereupon, the Spirit was hovering over the waters. "Much as would a potter's hands hover over the formless clay, in preparation for the task ahead. So, likewise, to solicit the interest of the listener in what would follow."[1]

The formula *God said* is used repeatedly in the first chapter of Genesis, as indicative of his sovereign power and creative disposition. As for the former, it is in the form of a mandate. As for the latter, it reflects God's innovative character. Consequently, it ought to not surprise us when he works in some unexpected manner.

And it was so or its equivalent is employed in response. As clay responds to the artisan's touch. In an orchestrated manner, each aspect of creation serves the harmonious whole. Were the Creator less precise, life as we know it would assuredly be impossible.

And God saw that it was good. In each instance, he then pronounced it *very good* (v. 31). It is *good* in the dual sense of being functional and aesthetically pleasing. Illustrative of the former, when one drinks a refreshing glass of water after laboring through the heat of the day. In regard to the latter, as when watching a waterfall cascading down sheer rock.

"What do you read concerning the creation of mankind?" the rabbi continued. He supposed this would be of critical importance.

"Then God said, 'Let us make man in our image, in our likeness,'" the student diligently responded, "'and let them rule over the fish of the sea and the birds of the air, over the livestock, over all the earth, and over all the creatures that move along the ground'" (v. 26). *Let us* appears to be a royal idiom,

---

1. Inch, *Scripture As Story*, 18.

still in use today—as were the monarch to say, "It seems to *us*" rather than "it appears to *me*."

In our image has been extrapolated in three connections. First, as expressive of a privileged ability to commune with one's Maker. In analogous terms, as a child would converse with its parents. Hence, regarding relatively simple matters.

Second, concerning the delegated authority to exercise stewardship over creation. This is in keeping with the maxim that God does not require us to do something which we are incapable of by his grace. It, in turn, recalls Mother Teresa's humorous observation: "I don't doubt that God will enable me to do his bidding, but I wished he were not so optimistic."

Finally, more specifically concerning the endowment for his unique role in the universe. Such as the ability to employ language so as to reflect back on the past, anticipate what will likely come to pass, and make wise decisions. Then, too, all that is associated with his rational, emotional, and volitional nature.

"So God created man in his own image, in the image of God he created him, male and female he created them" (v. 17). Thus are we alerted to the fact that the term *man* can be used either in a generic or inclusive sense. God also blessed them, and said: "Be fruitful and increase in number, fill the earth and subdue it." Conversely, he was not to ravage his environment.

"What else do you read?" the mentor shortly inquired. In proverbial terms, "He was not content to leave any stone unturned."

"By the seventh day God had finished the work he had been doing; so on the seventh day he rested from all his work," his protégé obediently replied. "And God blessed the seventh day and made it holy because on it he rested from all the work of creating that he had done" (2:2–3). From a rabbinic perspective:

> while it is certainly true that the Shabbat rejuvenates man's spirit, replenishes his physical strength, and revitalizes him so that he is able to face another work week, the deeper meaning of the Shabbat is that it is observed not for the sake of the rest of the week, but that the rest of the week is the prologue for the arrival of Sabbat[2]

Since it provides a means for sanctifying time. Moreover, in Jewish tradition it is customary to count toward the Sabbath: six days, five days, etc. This served to heighten one's anticipation, and make for a joyous celebration.

"Now the Lord God had planted a garden in the east, in Eden, and there he put the man he had formed. And the Lord God made all kinds of trees grow out of the ground—trees that were pleasing to the eye and good for food" (8–9). The imagery would be familiar to anyone acquainted with the Middle East. In particular, I recall walking in the garden in the cool of the day, after the oppressive heat earlier on. Then, too, of the pleasant assortment of trees and shrubbery. We would also gather from the text that there was ample provision.

"In the middle of the garden were the tree of life and the tree of the knowledge of good and evil." Whereas, the former would appear self-explanatory, the implications of the latter are more obscure. One is minimally assured that it pertains to moral discernment. However, it may also comprise a comprehensive idiom—similar to *as far as the east is from the west*;

---

2. Eckstein, *How Firm a Foundation*, 64.

and, if so, eating from it would imply that man meant to assert his autonomy. In addition, the garden was well watered.

Whereupon, the Lord God took the man and put him in the garden to tend it. And he commanded him, "You are free to eat from any tree in the garden; but you must not eat from the tree of the knowledge of good and evil, for when you eat of it you will surely die" (vv. 16–17), thereby losing access to the tree of life.

The Lord God also determined, "It is not good for the man to be alone. I will make a helper suitable for him." "Then the Lord God made a woman from the rib he had taken out of the man, and he brought her to the man." The man said, "This is now bone of my bones and flesh of my flesh; she shall be called 'woman,' for she was taken out of man." The writer then observes, "For this reason a man will leave his father and mother and be united to his wife, and they will become one flesh."

As for apt commentary,

> here the ideal of marriage as it was understood in ancient Israel is being portrayed a relationship characterized by harmony and intimacy between the partners. The destruction of this relationship is described in the following chapters, but like other aspects of man's existence set out in Gen. 1–2, the first days of the first marriage remain a goal to which Israel hoped to return when the promises to Abraham were fulfilled.[3]

---

3. Wenham, *Genesis 1–15*, 69.

In Jewish tradition, religious fidelity is realized primarily in a family context, as an indication of the importance attached to the home.

Not content with the discussion up to that point, the rabbi asked: "What do you read concerning man's fall?"

In response, the student cited how the serpent impugned God's veracity: "You will not surely die. For God knows that when you eat of it your eyes will be opened, and you will be like God, knowing good and evil" (3:4–5).

"When the woman saw that the fruit of the tree was good for food and pleasing to the eye, and also desirable for gaining wisdom, she took some and ate it. She also gave some to her husband, and he ate it." Then the eyes of both were opened, and they realized that they were naked; so that they sewed fig leaves together and made coverings for themselves. Their innocent serenity having been shattered, their action suggests urgency and desperation.

When they heard the sound of the Lord God walking in the garden, they hid themselves among the trees. Accordingly, the Almighty called out to them, "Where are you?" In this connection, we see God taking the initiative—a scenario repeated throughout the scriptures. It was this that solicited Francis Thompson's graphic description of the Almighty as the *Hound of Heaven*.

The Lord God subsequently inquired, "What is this that you have done?" (v. 13). It was in the way of enjoining them to consider the implications of their behavior, rather than being uninformed. In particular, that is in partaking of the forbidden fruit, they had violated the provisions of their implied covenant with the Almighty. Much as would an unappreciative child, who ignores its parent's wishes.

"The serpent deceived me," Eve replied. It was a partial truth at best, since she had been cautioned not to eat of the forbidden fruit. As a matter of fact, there was sufficient blame to go around.

Whereupon, the Lord addressed the serpent: "Cursed are you above all the livestock and all the wild animals. You will crawl on your belly and you will eat dust all the days of your life. And I will put enmity between you and the woman, and between your offspring and hers; he will crush your head, and you will strike his heel.

In this connection, the associated themes of struggle, suffering, and triumph are clearly set forth. There would be an ongoing struggle between the two adversaries, eventuating in prolonged suffering. However, the seed of woman would triumph in the end. This complex theme would come to mind when one saw a snake slithering along the ground, or coiled in preparation to strike its unsuspecting victim.

As mentioned earlier, God then informed Eve that the pain associated with birthing a child would be greatly increased. It is perhaps significant that he does not say that she would have been altogether without pain previously. It would, in any case, be much more tolerable and even welcomed in context of giving birth. Jesus observed in this connection, "A woman giving birth to a child has pain because her time has come; but when her baby is born she forgets the anguish because of her joy that a child is born into the world" (John 16:21).

As concerns Adam:

> Cursed is the ground because of you; through painful toil you will eat of it all the days of your life. It will produce thorns and thistles for you, and you

> will eat the plants of the field. By the sweat of your brow you will eat your food until you return to the ground, since from it you were taken; for dust you are and to dust you will return.

"The toil that now lies behind the preparation of every meal is a reminder of the fall and is made the more painful by the memory of the ready supply of food within the garden."[4]

So the Lord God banished them from paradise, lest they eat from the tree of life and perpetuate their fallen state. "After he drove the man out, he placed on the east side of the Garden of Eden cherubim and a flaming sword flashing back and forth to guard the way to the tree of life" (v. 24).

This imagery gave rise to John Milton's epic verse:

> They, looking back, all th' eastern side beheld
> Of Paradise, so late their happy seat,
> Waved over by the flaming brand; the gate
> With dreadful faces thronged and fiery arms
> Some natural tears they dropped, but wiped them soon;
> The world was all before them, where to choose
> Their place of rest, and Providence their guide.
> They, hand in hand, with wandering steps and slow,
> Through Eden took their solitary way.[5]

It was not the best of situations, but neither was it the worst. Granted, they had forfeited the gratifying accommodation of paradise, but God had not altogether absented himself. Or, as Milton expresses it, with *Providence their guide.*

"What are we to make of this narrative?" the elder audibly mused. The younger did not venture an answer, but respect-

---

4. Ibid., 82.
5. Milton, *Paradise Lost*, XII, 36–44.

fully deferred to his mentor. According to the sage, "There is a time to be silent and a time to speak" (Eccl 3:7). So it was that the lad perceived this was not a time to attempt a reply.

Initially, his mentor quoted from memory:

> Life is good. Wherefore a man should treasure it, not despise; affirm, and not deny it; have faith in it and never despair of its possibilities. For behind it is God. Life is good and man can find it such, provided—and this is the great condition to everything else, that it is properly lived.[6]

Ah, there is the rub: providing *it is lived properly*—according to God's directives.

As for a compelling rationale, since God is the author of life, it should be cherished. Not simply under ideal circumstances, but when qualified in some manner or another. One day at a time, along with the opportunities life affords us.

As a matter of concern, it seems that we are increasingly substituting a culture of death for a culture of life. As evidenced by the fact that we turn to violent means to achieve our several purposes, practice abortion for convenience, and lack civility in the public arena.

Secondly, we live from what may be described as *the middle*, between paradise lost and regained. As a result, we have difficulty identifying with both former and subsequent situations. Except, perhaps, in terms of an appropriate analogy. In this instance, as concerns a solicitous parent.

In greater detail, the parent prescribes the way the infant should behave. For instance, a child is told not to go out into

---

6. Steinberg, *Basic Judaism*, 59.

the road. Then, when older, he or she is told to look both ways before crossing.

Of course, the child might decide that the parents did not have its best interests at heart. This would not be unlike the disposition expressed by the original couple in partaking of the forbidden fruit. Then, too, with potentially disastrous results.

So we would conclude that life in paradise cultivated a blessed innocence. One that radiated confidence in the benevolent purposes of the Almighty, and zestfully went about one's duties. Consequently, maturing in the process.

As carried over into Jewish educational practice, the parent structures life to encourage the child to ask pertinent questions. Whereupon, he or she explains what is implicated by this or that. In deliberate manner, requiring seemingly endless patience and resolve (cf. Isa 28:10).

Thirdly, industry was encouraged. This serves as a means of fulfillment, growing out of a sense of calling. As would a steward, in anticipation of giving an accounting to his or her employer. Moreover, as an artisan, who takes satisfaction in doing some task well. Thus free from drudgery that often accompanies our labor from *the middle*, with paradise lost.

The ideal of industry is coupled in Jewish tradition with that of generosity. The rabbi surprisingly recalled a parable employed by Jesus. It seems that a certain rich man produced a good crop. "What shall I do?" he thought to himself. "I have no place to store my crops" (Luke 12:17). Accordingly, he decided to tear down his barns, and build larger ones—to accommodate a bumper crop. "And I will say to myself, 'You have plenty of good things laid up for many years. Take life easy; eat, drink and be merry.'" Consequently, he showed no regard for the needs of others—of whom there were many in the culture of that time.

"You fool!" God reprimanded him. "This very night your life will be demanded from you. Then who will get what you have prepared for yourself?" This is how it will be with anyone who stores up things for himself but is not rich toward God.

Fourthly, it is critical that we get our priorities in order. Consequently, to please God, even when disinclined to do so. Incidentally, the rabbis taught that it was more meritorious to obey when not so disposed. This takes on the form of *obedience*, since it renders him the honor due; and *trust*, because his ways are superior to our own.

Likewise, to consider the welfare of others along with our own, since both are legitimate concerns. Not given to extremes, thereby with disregard for one or the other. In that when we try to escape one fault, we are prone to fall prey to its opposite.

The rabbi now paused for effect, while his student continued to listen attentively. "Finally," the rabbi observed, "and this appears to be the crux of the issue, to recognize that the human potential for pain is commensurate with that of pleasure." The more of the one, the more of the other; the less of the one, the less of the other. In a manner of speaking, the stakes go up with humanity.

By way of illustration, the story is told of a group of devout Jews witnessing the destruction of the revered Temple. As one would expect, their anguish was expressed through weeping and wailing. However, one of their number seemed inexplicably joyful. When asked how he could rejoice on such an occasion, he replied: "If the razing of our beloved sanctuary results in such distress, imagine how great our rejoicing when it is rebuilt." Just so!

With such in mind, we are encouraged: "He makes the springs pour water into the ravines; it flows between the mountains. They give water to all the beasts of the field; the wild donkeys quench their thirst" (Ps 104:10–11). "As a freshwater spring in a semiarid land would be to a shepherd and his thirsty flock, so will be the eternal presence of God to redeemed humanity in their longing for spiritual wholeness."[7] Meanwhile, life resembles a journey to the celestial city. There are hardships to be creatively engaged, and pleasures to be thoroughly enjoyed. Not one to the exclusion of the other, since they are part of the same package. In any case, God's grace is abundant.

The elder spoke from experience, as he was nearing the end of his pilgrimage. As for the youth, his journey had only recently begun. Even so, he had received good counsel, and was the better for it.

---

7. Mounce, *The Book of Revelation*, 167.

2

The Sage

WE SOON encounter another inviting and revealing narrative. Job was an exceedingly devout person, overwhelmed by troubles. He is stripped of his wealth, family, and health. The cosmic struggle between good and evil plays out in the background, reminding us that there is more involved than meets the eye.

Three *friends* try to console him in his suffering. However, each seems to have a personal agenda. Subsequently, a fourth joins them, but adds little of constructive value. "Eventually the Lord Himself addresses Job. These speeches change Job's attitude, for he responds with contrite submission. In the end God declares Job to be in the right and restores his prosperity and happiness."[1]

In greater detail, "In the land of Uz there lived a man whose name was Job. This man was blameless and upright; he feared God and shunned evil" (Job 1:1). For a person living west of the great rift valley, anything across the Jordan River would be categorized as the *east*. "It was not desert, for in fertile places there could be tillage and towns, at least in good times. Here could be seen both nomadic shepherd and settled

---

1. Anderson, *Job*, 15.

farmer; and sometimes the same person could be both."[2] Here the patriarch Job lived and prospered.

His demeanor greatly pleased the Almighty. Now it came to pass that the angels came to present themselves before the Lord God, and Satan also came with them. Whereupon, the Sovereign Lord inquired of Satan, "Have you considered my servant Job? There is no one on earth like him; he is blameless and upright, a man who fears God and shuns evil" (v. 8).

"Does Job fear God for nothing?" the adversary replied. "Have you not put a hedge around him and his household and everything he has? You have blessed the work of his hands, so that his flocks and herds are spread throughout the land. But stretch out your hand and strike everything he has, and he will surely curse you to your face."

"Very well, then," the Lord responded, "everything he has is in your hands, but on the man himself do not lay a finger." One day a messenger came to Job with the disconcerting news: "The oxen were plowing and the donkeys were grazing nearby, and the Sabeans attacked and carried them off. They put the servants to the sword, and I am the only one who has escaped to tell you!" (vv. 14–15).

While he was speaking, another messenger came and said: "The fire of God fell from the sky and burned up the sheep and the servants, and I am the only one who has escaped to tell you!"

While he was speaking, yet another messenger arrived and said: "The Chaldeans formed three raiding parties and swept down on your camels and carried them off. They put the servants to the sword, and I am the only one who has escaped to tell you!"

2. Ibid., 77.

While he was speaking, a final messenger put in an appearance, saying: "Your sons and daughters were feasting and drinking wine at the oldest brother's house, when suddenly a mighty wind swept in from the desert and struck the four corners of the house. It collapsed on them and they are dead, and I am the only one who has escaped to tell you!"

At this, the patriarch struggled to his feet, tore his robe, and shaved his head—as a sign of mourning. Whereupon, he prostrated himself, acknowledging: "Naked I came from my mother's womb, and naked I will depart. The Lord gave and the Lord has taken away; may the name of the Lord be praised." "In all this," the chronicler appreciatively observes, "Job did not sin by charging God with wrongdoing."

On another day the angels came to present themselves before the Lord, and Satan was again with them. "Have you considered my servant Job?" the Lord again asks of him. "There is no one on earth like him, he is blameless and upright, a man who fears God and shuns evil. And he still maintains his integrity, although you incited me against him to ruin him without any reason" (2:3).

"Skin for skin!" Satan exclaims. "A man will give all he has for his own life. But stretch out your hand and strike his flesh and bones, and he will surely curse you to your face." He appears determined to undermine the patriarch's integrity.

"Very well, then," the Lord allowed, "he is in your hands, but you must spare his life." This should demonstrate Job's integrity beyond a shadow of a doubt.

So it was that the adversary afflicted Job with painful sores from the sole of his feet to the top of his head. Then the patriarch took a piece of broken pottery, and scraped himself with it as he sat among the ashes. The reference is likely to the rubbish dump outside the city, perhaps indicating that he was an outcast.

"Are you still holding to your integrity?" his wife incredulously inquires. "Curse God and die!" Perhaps she had given up on God, and thinks her husband should do the same. In any case, she would like to see him out of his misery.

> We can readily appreciate the wife's feeling for we, too, are often tempted to reach the same conclusion. A particularly trying experience comes along and we back off, sulk away from God, shirk our responsibilities, and become embittered with life. We fail to see the development as part of God's providential plan and a means to help us reap the rich bounty of life.[3]

"You are talking like a foolish woman," Job protests. "Shall we accept good from God, and not trouble?" "In all this," the chronicler again observes, "Job did not sin in what he said."

When Job's *three friends* (Eliphaz the Temanite, Bildad the Shuhite, and Zophar the Naamathite) "heard about all the troubles that had come upon him, they set out from their homes and met by agreement to go and sympathize with him and comfort him" (v. 11). The prior basis for their friendship is not mentioned, but their diverse backgrounds serve as a reminder of Job's prominence in the region.

When they saw the patriarch from a distance, they could hardly recognize him. They began to weep aloud, rent their robes, and sprinkled dust on their heads. Then they sat on the ground with him for seven days and seven nights. *Seven days* was the statuatory period for mourning the dead, but this may

---

3. Inch, *My Servant Job*, 26.

simply be idiomatic for an extended or proper period of time. "No one said a word to him, because they saw how great his suffering was." In particular, it was compounded by his painful malady, social alienation, loss of family and associates, and the feeling of being forsaken in his time of dire need.

Job subsequently broke the silence. "May the day of my birth perish," he vented. "That day, may it turn to darkness; may God above not care about it; may no light shine upon it" (3:1–2).

Then Eliphaz ventured a reply.

> According to (him), Job had grown callous in the midst of riches and allowed unrighteousness to creep into his life. The misfortune befalling him was God's judgment, a warning to mend his ways. Job could either turn from his sin and be restored to divine favor or persist in his evil and anticipate the continuing heavy hand of God.[4]

Job asked for a bill of particulars. "Teach me, and I will be silent; and show me how I have erred" (6:24). Otherwise, no simplistic solution would suffice. Especially one that failed to take into consideration the ambiguity that permeates life.

Every so often one hears the complaint, "Why did this happen to me?" Probably not for any reason we can readily identify. Such as some illness arbitrarily inflicted as a punishment. Granted, in a larger sense, our misbehavior is calculated to adversely effect us, but there is seldom a simple correlation.

Learning to live with ambiguity does not mean assuming a passive roll. Quite the reverse! It helps us ask the hard

---

4. Ibid., 39.

questions, even though the answers come with difficulty. It also presses us to take responsible action, although we do so with care. Consequently, Job rightly demanded specifics as a guide to corrective action.

Consider the interchange from a different perspective. Eliphaz had God neatly packaged, and eminently predictable. As a result, he could be readily manipulated.

Conversely, the patriarch recognized that God works in mysterious ways, in keeping with the realization: "As the heavens are higher than the earth, so are my (God's) ways than your ways and my thoughts than your thoughts" (Isa 55:9). This, in turn, recalls the psalmist's rejoinder: "When I consider your heavens, the work of your fingers, the moon and the stars, which you have set in place, what is man that you are mindful of him, the son of man that you care for him?" (8:3–4). In this regard, we are reminded of God's benevolent concern.

If the patriarch did not have it bad enough, he had to put up with Eliphaz's incrimination. In a manner of speaking, the latter waved his finger under Job's nose, instead of putting an arm around his shoulders. In contrast, "A friend loves at all times, and a brother is born for adversity" (Prov 17:17).

One wonders about Eliphaz's peculiar insensitivity. Perhaps Job's calamity alarmed him concerning his own vulnerability. If disaster could so quickly befall the patriarch, he might be next in line. Unless, that is, he would demonstrate his virtue by insisting on Job's defection. One cannot say for certain.

In contrast, "Job saw life for what it is, a place where situations are difficult to diagnose, solutions are problematic, God's working is mysterious, and people are a mixture of good and bad."[5] Moreover, he embraced life in these terms, and in the end, he was commended.

"Ask from the former generations and find out what their fathers learned," Bildad subsequently counsels, "for we were born only yesterday and know nothing, and our days on earth are but a shadow" (8:8–9). Since we can only draw superficial conclusions from fleeting impressions, tradition provides the more trustworthy guide.

"Indeed" Job admits, "I know that this is true, but how can a mortal be righteous before God?" (9:1). History never simply repeats itself, so that we must apply abiding truths to changing circumstances. So while we ought to learn from the past, we ought not to become enslaved to it.

Then, too, tradition combines the bad with the good. While we can learn from both, it is necessary to sort out the different elements. Even then, there may be complex features that we overlook.

Much of the interchange focuses on what constitutes *obligation*; that is, what is involved in being faithful to one's tradition. It seems obvious that Bildad approaches this in a rigid, uncompromising fashion, while Job sees it as a more dynamic process. As for the patriarch, it is an approach that allows for a creative application.

"If you say, 'how we will hound him, since the root of the trouble lies in him,'" Job pointedly concludes, "you should fear the sword yourselves, for wrath will bring punishment by the sword, and then you will know that there is judgment" (19:28–29). In other words, "For in the same way you judge others, you will be judged, and with the measure you use, it will be measured to you" (Matt 7:2).

5. Ibid., 49.

"Zophar's brashly announced that God had exacted less from Job than his guilt deserved (11:6) and followed up this presumptive charge with a clear distortion of the patriarch's behavior (20:18–21). His prejudice drips with each succeeding comment."[6] Then, too, in a confrontational manner, so as to coerce submission.

No doubt the writer means to imply that there is something of Zophar in all of us. How then are we to deal with it? We must first realize that there are often good reasons why people disagree with us. In this connection, life resembles a circle of people surveying a painting. One sees one thing, and someone else sees something different. As a result, they interpret the remainder in terms of that which impressed them most.

Are all the views equally valid? Decidedly not! However, some people have a better grasp of reality than others. As a rule, this is gained as one matures—although some make better use of their experience than others. Nothing is achieved by repeating the same mistake over and over again.

Since the preponderance of what we embrace as true is derived from others, we ought to select our mentors carefully. In general, we should defer to those with informed insight in the appropriate discipline. For instance, one should not turn to a casual observer in preference to one who has carefully weighed the issues. Nor should one assume that an economist is the best guide in matters dealing with astronomy.

All things considered, life is too rich to be viewed from a narrow, partisan perspective. As expressed by Augustine, "All truth is God's truth." Hence, one's convictions should be open

---

6. Ibid., 64.

to modification, in the light of further evidence. Zophar's appeal, consequently, left much to be desired.

The three men stopped answering Job, since he perceived himself not at fault for that which had happened to him. Elihu, however, not only took issue with him, but was distressed that the others had failed in their attempt to convince Job. "I am still young in years," he admits, "and you are old; that is why I was fearful, not daring to tell you what I know" (32:6). Still, he supposes that God distributes wisdom as he wills.

Elihu mentions four times being angry over the stalemate between Job and his accusers. As a result, he appears driven by anger to throw caution to the wind. "My words come from an upright heart," he assures the patriarch, "my lips sincerely speak what I know" (33:3).

The issue of credibility enters with Elihu. "No one should doubt the necessity of having faith. To negotiate life at all, we must believe in something, somehow. We cannot choose whether to believe, but we must decide among the vast array of possibilities presented for our consideration."[7]

Faith, as exercised by the patriarch, implies taking God at his word, and acting upon it. Some convictions strain under the weight of contrary evidence until they collapse. Others seem refined in the crucible of life until they become strong and durable. Job's faith is of the latter sort.

Elihu proposes to speak for the Almighty, and condemns the patriarch in the process. "Earlier Job's irreverence was attributed to stupidity rather than to wickedness. The former might be cured by instruction in wisdom. The cure

---

7. Ibid., 76.

of the latter is more difficult, especially when it is willful and repeated."[8]

The accuser dangled his religious certainties before Job, but the patriarch refused to bite. The tempting lure meant to drag him into credulity, to put fiction in place of fact. In this manner, cultivating uncritical commitment to an improvised deity. Conversely, an untroubled confidence may not qualify as genuine.

The Lord subsequently spoke to Job out of the storm. This was calculated to reassure the patriarch.

Job stands out as a paragon of virtue. We were alerted to this at the outset. However, in the light of God's awesome presence, he earnestly repents of his presumption to pontificate on things of which he had little knowledge.

After the Lord had spoken with Job, he turned to Eliphaz. "I am angry with you and your two friends, because you have not spoken of me what is right, as my servant Job has" (42:7). Consequently, he was enjoined to offer a sacrifice, with the assurance that the patriarch would intercede on their behalf. "After Job had prayed for his friends, the Lord made him prosperous again and gave him twice as much as he had before" (v. 16).

In answer to the question concerning why the godly suffer, three prime considerations surface. First, God is deserving of our approval apart from the blessings he abundantly bestows. As one who is righteous in all his ways, and eminently wise.

In this connection, Jesus taught his disciples to pray: "Our Father in heaven, hallowed be your name" (Matt 6:9). The notion of *father* in Semitic thought primarily conveys the

8. Anderson, *op. cit.*, 255.

notion of deserving authority. In keeping with God's exalted position, we are enjoined to give him due honor, and not diminish it by entertaining false deities (cf. Exod 20:2).

Second, divine omnipotence is manifest through bringing good out of suffering. Not as some suppose, as an evidence of its lack. In the light of this realization, we do well to embrace suffering as a means to refine our spiritual devotion.

Even so, God is more disposed to use incentives than retribution. This is brought out in Job's earlier and later experience, between which he is sorely tested. This is graphically described by C. S. Lewis as a preference for *carrots* rather than *clubs*. As for the former, it more often resembles a whisper. As the latter, it can come as a shout. Only on relatively rare occasions does God lift his voice.

Finally, "As the heavens are higher than the earth, so are my ways higher than your ways and my thoughts higher than your thoughts," says the Almighty (Isa 55:9). Not simply because of his comprehensive understanding, but due to his moral purity. It goes without saying that sin distorts reality.

So it is that God's ways often appear quite mysterious to us. Most so initially, and sometimes less so as we look back on the way the Lord has led us. No doubt this testifies to his remarkable creativity.

3

The Passion Legacy

THE PASSION narratives play a distinctive role in exploring the realm of suffering. Luke, as an example, touches in passing on Jesus' early life, elaborates more extensively concerning his public ministry, and dwells at much greater length on Jesus' passion. In particular, the *passion* documents Jesus' suffering in the course of realizing his redemptive calling.

"He (Jesus) then (having been identified as the Messiah) began to teach them (his disciples) that the Son of Man (with reference to himself) must suffer many things and be rejected by the elders, chief priests and teachers of the law, and that he must be killed and after three days rise again" (Mark 8:31). Whereupon, Peter took him aside, and began to rebuke him. "Get behind me, Satan!" Jesus exclaimed. "You do not have in mind the things of God, but the things of men."

Jesus had previously been more guarded in his remarks, but now speaks openly.

> The comment that Jesus was speaking the word openly indicates the decisive character of this incident in the context of Jesus' persistent use of veiled, parabolic speech. Peter's reaction shows that it was impossible to miss what Jesus intended to say, even

though the divine necessity for his suffering appeared inconceivable."[1]

Jesus, in turn, reveals no compulsion to justify God's ways to human predilection. As if to suggest that there is no resolution to the human dilemma which precludes the need for suffering. In other words, grace proves to be costly. Initially, for Jesus; and subsequently, for his disciples.

Jesus then summoned the crowd to hear his extended commentary. Whereupon, he said to them: "If anyone would come after me, he must deny himself and take up his cross and follow me. For whoever wants to save his life will lose it, but whoever loses his life for me and for the gospel will save it."

> Jesus' words envision men before a court where denial of association with him will bring release while affirmation of "Jesus and the gospel" issues in martyrdom. He thoroughly appreciates the frailty of human life threatened by death, but warns that the man who seeks to secure his own existence by denial of his Lord brings about his own destruction.[2]

"What good is it for man to gain the whole world, yet forfeit his soul?" he rhetorically inquires. "Or what can a man give in exchange for his soul?" Which brings to mind the death of a certain affluent person. "How much did he leave?" one person curiously inquired.

"So far as I know," his companion replied, "all of it." Consequently, it bears repeating: "What good is it for a man to gain the whole world, yet forfeit his soul?"

1. Lane, *The Gospel of Mark*, 303.
2. Ibid., 308.

"If anyone is ashamed of me and my words in this adulterous and sinful generation," Jesus pointedly continued, "the Son of Man will be ashamed of him when he comes in his Father's glory with the holy angels." This reference to *his Father's glory with the holy angels* serves to frame Jesus' ministry in context of a doxology. Then, too, it is set over against the human tendency for self-emulation.

Of course, Jesus encountered pain long before his formidable passion experience. Two examples will suffice to illustrate. Early in his public ministry, he returned to Nazareth—where he was raised. As was his custom, he made his way to the synagogue on the Sabbath. He stood up to read, and the Isaiah scroll was handed to him.

Unrolling it, he found the place where it was written: "The Spirit of the Lord is on me, because he has anointed me to preach the good news to the poor. He has sent me to proclaim freedom for the prisoners and recovery of sight for the blind, to release the oppressed, to proclaim the year of the Lord's favor" (Luke 4:18–19; cf. Isa 61:1–2). He stopped pointedly short of an allusion to judgment. It consisted of Jubilee imagery appropriate for the Messianic Age.

Then he rolled up the scroll, gave it back to the attendant, and sat down—the customary manner assumed in teaching. The eyes of everyone in the synagogue were fixed on him, and he began by saying: "Today this scripture is fulfilled in your hearing."

The people were amazed at the *gracious words* that came from his mouth, and inquired: "Isn't this Joseph's son?" We would gather from this that they associated nothing unusual with Jesus from his childhood and youth. Unlike later accounts which attributed to him such things as creating clay birds, and giving them life.

"Surely you will quote this proverb to me," Jesus observed: "'Physician, heal yourself! Do here in your home-town what we have heard that you did in Capernaum.'" "I tell you the truth," he continued,

> no prophet is accepted in his home-town. I assure that there were many widows in Israel in Elijah's time, when the sky was shut for three and a half years and there was a severe famine throughout the land. Yet Elijah was not sent to any of them, but to a widow in Zarephath in the region of Sidon. And there were many in Israel with leprosy in the time of Elisha the prophet, yet not one of them was cleansed—only Naaman the Syrian.

All those in attendance were furious when they heard this, and drove him out of town to the brow of the hill on which the town was built, meaning to cast him down the cliff. As a relevant aside, Capernaum was frequented by Gentiles, since it was located on a branch of the *Via Maris* (international trade route), while Nazareth was much more secluded. Consequently, the people objected to the idea that God would show his favor to Gentiles in preference to his chosen people.

However, Jesus walked through the crowd, and went on his way. Luke does not reveal how this was possible. If it was a miracle, it was decidedly not the kind that the people had hoped to see Jesus perform. In any case, this must have been an exceedingly painful experience for Jesus, having been rejected by those with whom he had grown to maturity, and with whom he recalled many enjoyable occasions.

The second incident occurs later on in Jesus' public ministry. He characterized himself as *the bread of life*. Many of his disciples concluded that this was a difficult saying to embrace. From this time many of his disciples turned back, and no longer followed him. "Until his refusal to be made their king, they had heard him gladly, but when he put them off by his insistence on the superiority of the bread of eternal life ... they lost interest. What they wanted, he would not give; what he offered, they would not receive."[3]

"You do not want to leave too, do you?" Jesus plaintively asked the Twelve (John 6:67). One can readily sense in his words the hurt accompanying the loss of his previous disciples. One would hope that the Twelve would not follow suit, since that would greatly intensify the painful separation.

"Lord, to whom shall we go?" Peter inquired. "You have the words of eternal life. We believe and know that you are the Holy One of God." We would gather that he meant to speak on behalf of the others; only Judas would defect.

Now Jesus eventually made his way up to Jerusalem. When he came near to the place where the road goes down the Mount of Olives, the whole crowd of disciples began joyfully to praise God in loud voices for all the miracles they had seen; "Blessed is the king who comes in the name of the Lord! Peace in heaven and glory in the highest!" (Luke 19:38).

"Teacher," some of the Pharisees in the crowd implored Jesus, "rebuke your disciples!"

"I tell you," he replied, "if they keep quiet, the stones will cry out." It was likely a proverbial saying, perhaps derived from the notion of piling stones as a witness.

---

3. Bruce, *The Gospel of John*, 164.

As Jesus approached the city, he wept over it. "If you, even you, had only known on this day what would bring you peace—but now it is hidden from your eyes," he solemnly reflected.

> The days will come upon you when your enemies will build an embankment against you and encircle you and hem you in on every side. They will dash you to the ground, you and the children within your walls. They will not leave one stone on another, because you did not recognize the time of God's coming to you.

Consequently, it is not surprising that he wept over the beloved City of the Great King.

After Jesus had eaten the last supper with his disciples, they went out to the Mount of Olives. "Pray that you will not fall into temptation," he urged them. Then, after with-drawing about a stone's throw, he petitioned: "Father, if you are willing, take this cup from me; yet not my will, but yours be done" (Luke 22:42). Jesus is keenly aware of the suffering that awaits him, and would prefer an alternative course—were it in keeping with his Father's will. Instead, an angel appeared to strengthen him in his resolve.

"And being in anguish, he prayed more earnestly, and his sweat was like drops of blood falling to the ground." In what manner did it resemble blood? Alexander Metherell speculates in this regard:

> This is a known medical condition called hematidrosis. It's not very common, but it is associated with a high degree of psychological stress. What happens is that severe anxiety causes the release

> of chemicals that break down the capillaries in the sweat glands. As a result, there's a small amount of bleeding into these glands, and the sweat comes out tinged with blood.[4]

In any case, Luke means to assure us that Jesus was experiencing extreme anguish in anticipation of his imminent demise.

Thus are we alerted to the fact that suffering occurs in anticipation of some undesirable experience, during it, and upon reflection. Jesus was in the initial stage of the passion narrative, which served to prime him for what would follow. If one accepts the prior reconstruction, this would have physical ramifications—since Jesus' condition would have made his skin more sensitive to his subsequent flogging.

When Jesus rose from prayer, he found his disciples fast asleep—*exhausted from sorrow.* "Why are you sleeping?" he asked them. "Get up and pray so that you will not fall into temptation." Along with this came the realization that he had maintained the prayer vigil alone.

While he was yet speaking, a crowd engulfed them—led by Judas, pointedly identified as *one of the Twelve.* "Judas," Jesus reproached him, "are you betraying the Son of Man with a kiss?"

"Lord," Jesus' disciples inquired, "should we strike with our swords?" Peter did not wait for an answer, but struck a servant of the high priest—cutting off his ear. "No more of this!" Jesus exclaimed. He then touched the man's ear and healed him.

They seized him, and led him away to the house of the high priest. Peter followed at a discreet distance. The others

---

4. Strobel, *The Case For Christ*, 195.

appear to have fled. Peter would eventually deny him, as Jesus had anticipated.

Jesus appeared before the high priest, Pilate, and Herod. In each instance, in threatening circumstances. "I find no basis for a charge against this man," Pilate concluded (Luke 23:4). His accusers insisted that Jesus constituted a political threat, a charge that Pilate had to take seriously.

He subsequently had Jesus flogged.

> Roman floggings were known to be terribly brutal. They usually consisted of thirty-nine lashes but frequently were a lot more than that, depending on the mood of the soldier applying the blows. (He) would use a whip of braided leather thongs with metal balls woven into them. When the whip would strike the flesh these balls would cause deep bruises or contusions, which would break open with further blows.[5]

The whip might also have sharp pieces of bone attached, further intensifying the painful ordeal. This, in turn, was sometimes referred to as *a half-way death*, since the point was to bring the victim to death's threshold. While Jesus survived the abuse, it left him in critical condition.

The soldiers then proceeded to add insult to injury. Stripping him and putting a scarlet robe on him, they then twisted together a crown of thorns and set it on his head. They put a staff in his right hand and knelt in front of him and mocked him. "Hail, king of the Jews!" they said. The soldiers spit on him, and took the staff and struck him on the head again and again (Matt 27:28–30).

5. Ibid.

The Passion Legacy 33

They then led him away to be crucified. What did this initially entail? "He would have been laid down, and his hands would have been nailed in the outstretched position to the horizontal beam. This crossbar was called the patibulum, and at this stage it was separate from the vertical beam, which was permanently set in the ground."[6] The Romans employed spikes five to seven inches long, and were driven through the wrists.

Once a person is hung in a vertical position, crucifixion is characteristically an agonizingly slow death by asphyxiation, since the person must extend his body in order to exhale, until no longer able to do so. In Jesus' weakened condition, death came mercifully more quickly.

From the sixth to the ninth hour (noon to three p.m.) there was darkness over all the land. About the ninth hour, Jesus cried out: "My God, my God, why have you forsaken me?" (Matt 27:46; cf. Ps 22:1). His quote was from a psalm traditionally employed by those suffering affliction. Not to be overlooked, the text concludes on a positive note: "Posterity will serve him; future generations will be told about the Lord. They will proclaim his righteousness to a people yet unborn—for he has done it (fulfilled his promises)."

Jesus subsequently announced, "It is finished" (John 19:30). With this, he bowed his head and gave up his spirit. This marked not only the conclusion of his earthly sojourn, but the completion of the task that was entrusted to him. He had remained resolute throughout.

The passion narrative left a lasting impression on Jesus' disciples. In this regard, they would recall an observation cited

---

6. Ibid., 197.

earlier: "If anyone would come after me, he must deny himself and take up his cross and follow me" (Matt 16:24).

> To deny oneself—indeed to die to oneself—this is what it means to "follow" Jesus. In contrast to the preceding aorist imperatives, this verb is in the present tense, suggesting the ongoing practice of following. Thus the revelation of Jesus' own imminent suffering and death in the preceding pericope is now seen to be full of significance for the disciples themselves.[7]

The disciples were not allowed to choose the conditions under which they would suffer.

> While it is easier to suffer honorably and to the acclaim of others, they were not assured this would be the case. While it is easier to suffer with others than alone, they were not guaranteed this option. While perhaps easier to accept martyrdom than live as those who have died in Christ, the choice would be made for them.[8]

Weigh the implications of Jesus' words. Initially, he points out the voluntary character of discipleship. Should a person desire to follow him, then such and such pertains. Otherwise, the circumstances do not necessarily apply.

The alternative is not inviting. Life readily degenerates into the survival of the fittest. Justice is circumvented, and the strong prey on the weak. Even good intentions give way to pragmatic accommodations.

---

7. Hagner, *Matthew 14–28*, 483.

8. Inch, *Exhortations of Jesus According to Matthew* and *Up From the Depths*, 114.

Subsequently, discipleship involves self-denial. There are no exceptions, only varying circumstances. Otherwise expressed, this involves the crucifixion of the autonomous self—that which lives for selfish interests, regardless of the needs and concerns of others.

In this connection, we are disposed to accept the lesser good. In other words, all that falls short of God's purpose for our lives, and often used as an excuse for our lack of responsiveness. Such as is not uncommonly meant to solicit the praise of others, while falling critically short of divine acceptance.

In addition, discipleship anticipates suffering—as implied by taking up our cross. It is sometimes of physical character, as with Jesus' flogging and crucifixion. It is more often along the line of emotional stress, or some combination of the two.

Illustrations can be readily multiplied. A former classmate gathered that God would have him serve in West Africa. He accepted this challenge in good spirits. However, he soon died from a tropical disease—cutting short a promising ministry.

One of my students felt impressed to undertake a pioneer inner city ministry. It meant that he had to improvise, and deal with excessive uncertainty. While it took a toll, he was not dissuaded.

Whether in this context or some other, discipleship also involves the resolute determination to follow Jesus. In the face of formidable obstacles, when forsaken by others, and regardless of waning resolve. In terms of a gospel chorus, "I have decided to follow Jesus; no turning back, no turning back."

Not to be overlooked, discipleship also operates in the context of community. The individual Christian is an anomaly, since when we make our way to the cross, we discover others knelt there. Consequently, Dietrich Bonhoeffer supposes that it is very unlikely that one would ever fail to experience the fellowship of believers.

In brief, this involves being there for others, allowing them to be there for us, and open to God's initiatives. In this regard, Paul enjoins: "Carry each other's burdens, and in so doing you will fulfill the law of Christ" (Gal 6:2). Then, in paradoxical fashion, "each one should carry his own load"—since in shouldering our own burdens we do not become an unnecessary burden to others. Accordingly, we ought not to expect others to do for us what we are unwilling to do for ourselves.

All things considered, suffering serves as a refining agent. While it ought not to be solicited unnecessarily, it should be embraced in the context of God's providential design—in that it provides an unique opportunity for spiritual growth and related service.

So it can be seen that the long shadow of the cross extends throughout succeeding generations. It reminds us of Jesus' sacrifice on our behalf, and the invitation to participate in his suffering. This is set over against two alternatives. First, the temptation to escape—whether given a religious rationale or some other. Second, the attempt to engage the world on its own terms—apart from drawing on our abundant spiritual resources. So life would appear in the light of the memorable and provocative passion narrative.

4

Voices of the Martyrs

THE MARTYR provides a distinct perspective on suffering. Incidentally, the terrorist is not worthy of inclusion, since death is self-inflicted—along with the demise of others. We will consider three examples: Stephen, Ignatius, and Polycarp by way of getting a better handle on suffering in the context of martyrdom.

At a time when the numbers of disciples were increasing, a problem arose concerning the distribution of food to the fledgling congregation. In particular, the *Grecian Jews* complained that their widows were being overlooked. So the Twelve gathered the disciples together, and informed them: "It would not be right for us to neglect the ministry of the word of God in order to wait on tables. Brothers, choose seven men from among you who are known to be full of the Spirit and wisdom. We will turn this responsibility over to them" (Acts 6:2–3).

As for commentary, "The Hellenists of this passage were Christians drawn from the Greek-speaking synagogues of Jerusalem, and forming their own Greek-speaking community. . . . The apostles themselves were, of course, Hebrews."[1] So the neglect presumably was not intentional.

1. Williams, *Acts*, 118

Stephen was the first of the seven mentioned, and depicted as a person *full of faith and the Holy Spirit.* Hence, he was eminently qualified for the task to which the seven were appointed.

"Now Stephen, a man full of God's grace and power, did great wonders and miraculous signs among the people." This could be expected to increase his esteem in the community. Opposition arose, however, from members of the Synagogue of the Freedman (as it was called), consisting of Jews of Cyrene, Alexandria, and the provinces of Cilicia and Asia. That is to say, from among the Hellenistic Jews. "These began to argue with Stephen, but they could not stand up against the wisdom or the Spirit by whom he spoke."

So they stirred up the people, their elders, and the rabbis. Stephen was seized, and brought before the Sanhedrin—as the supreme religious council. False witnesses were solicited to testify that Stephen continually spoke against the temple and the law: "For we have heard him say that this Jesus of Nazareth will destroy the place and change the customs Moses handed down to us."

The members of the Sanhedrin looked intently at Stephen, whose face took on the likeness of an angel. Whereupon, the high priest pointedly inquired whether these charges were true.

"Brothers and fathers, listen to me!"—inviting their thoughtful consideration. "The God of glory appeared to our father Abraham while he was still in Mesopotamia, before he lived in Haran. 'Leave your country and your people,' God said, 'and go to the land I will show you'" (7:2–3). After that, he covenanted with the patriarch.

Later on, God "gave Joseph wisdom and enabled him to gain the goodwill of Pharaoh king of Egypt, so he made him ruler over Egypt and all his palace." As a consequence, the Israelites were subsequently able to find sanctuary.

Still later, God raised up Moses to deliver his people from bondage. This, too, came to pass. It was this Moses who promised the Israelites, "God will send you a prophet like me from your own people." Which, in turn, was the issue at hand.

However, the people were blatantly disobedient, invoking God's wrath. "You are just like your fathers," Stephen summarily accused them. "You always resist the Holy Spirit! Was there ever a prophet your fathers did not persecute? They even killed those who predicted the coming of the Righteous One. And now you have betrayed and murdered him."

When they heard this, they were furious with him. Conversely, Stephen being full of the Holy Spirit and gazing upward, declared: "I see heaven open and the Son of Man standing at the right hand of God." At this, the people covered their ears and shouting at the top of their voices, dragged him out of the city and began to stone him.

While being stoned, Stephen earnestly prayed: "Lord Jesus, receive my spirit." Then he fell on his knees and cried out: "Lord, do not hold this sin against them." Having said this, he fell asleep. Saul was there, giving assent to the martyr's death.

On that day, a great persecution broke out against the church at Jerusalem, and the believers were scattered throughout Judea and Samaria. Godly men buried Stephen, and mourned for him. Meanwhile, Saul set out to utterly destroy the community of faith. Although in time he would become the select apostle (Paul) to the Gentiles; and then, if the tradition is accurate, he would likewise suffer martyrdom.

Others would follow over the course of time. In particular, we turn our attention to Ignatius. In this regard:

> When Trajan, not long since, succeeded to the empire of the Romans (AD 98), Ignatius, the disciple of John the apostle, a man in all respects of an apostolic character, governed the Church of the Antiochians with great care, having with difficulty escaped the former storms of the many persecutions under Domitian, inasmuch as, like a good pilot, by the helm of prayer and fasting, by the earnestness of his teaching, and by his spiritual labor, he resisted the flood that rolled against him, fearing lest he should lose of those who were deficient in courage, or apt to suffer from their simplicity.[2]

Antioch was a prominent city, said by Josephus to be superceded only by Rome and Alexandria. It embraced from the outset a mixed population. "This mix of cultures had good and bad results. It gave rise, on the one hand, to the literature and art that won Antioch the praise of Cicero, but, on the other, to the luxury and immorality that made the disintegration of Roman morality."[3] This would require of Ignatius all the energy and wisdom at his command to shepherd his congregation.

In retrospect, the church at Antioch was founded early on by some who fled the persecution following Stephen's demise. It would eventually boast an impressive group of prophets and teachers; who, at the prompting of the Spirit, set apart

2. *The Martyrdom of Ignatius*, I.
3. Williams, *op. cit.*, 203.

Paul and Barnabas for their first missionary journey (cf. Acts 13:1–3).

Ignatius composed seven extant epistles while in transit from Antioch to Rome, where he would suffer martyrdom. These fall into two groups, written at different junctures along the way. The letters to the Ephesians, Magnesians, Trallians, and Romans were sent from Smyrna—while Ignatius was in personal contact with bishop Polycarp of that city. The remaining epistles (to the Philadelphians, Smyrnaeans, and Polycarp) were dispatched at a later juncture. We shall touch on select instances which illustrate his disposition toward suffering martyrdom.

Initially, "For even though I am in bonds for his Name's sake, I am not yet perfected in Jesus Christ."[4] He thus gives the impression of a work in progress. Once associated with his ministry at Antioch, now concerning his incarceration, and eventually with his martyrdom. Each succeeding stage is calculated to prepare him for the one to follow.

Given this perspective, we learn through the vicissitudes of life how to manage suffering. First in one connection, and then in another. Then, if called upon to experience martyrdom, to do so with passionate commitment.

In a later connection, "Remember me in your prayers, that I may attain unto God; and remember also the church which is in Syria, whereof I am not worthy to be called a member."[5] *Remember me in your prayers*, since they are effective means of grace. Then, too, they appear as a natural response to trying circumstances. Moreover, it is a practice best cultivated prior to adversity.

4. Ignatius, *To the Ephesians*, 3.
5. Ignatius, *To the Magnesians*, 14.

First, that *I may attain unto God*. In this regard, that he might rise to the occasion. Not as certain others, who repudiate their faith when threatened with reprisal. In brief, exercising confident courage.

Second, concerning the church in Syria. While commended for its faithfulness, it was still in need of prayerful support. Then, in turn, drawing strength from the intercession of fellow believers.

In a revealing text, "For though I desire to suffer, yet I know not whether I am worthy: for the envy of the devil is unseen indeed by many, but against me it wages the fiercer war. So then I crave gentleness, whereby the prince of this world is brought to naught."[6] His desire *to suffer* thus appears to derive from two sources: in that it consummated the process of sanctification in his own life, and because it serves as an encouragement to others.

He is, moreover, alert to the spiritual battle that he continues to wage with the evil adversary. Such as requires that he cultivate the Christian virtues in order to gain the victory. Consequently, not presuming that which has yet to be determined.

As concerns priorities, "It is good for me to die for Jesus Christ rather than to reign over the farthest bounds of the earth."[7] "What is more," Paul earnestly writes, "I consider everything loss compared to the surpassing greatness of knowing Christ Jesus my Lord, for whose sake I have lost all things. I consider them rubbish, that I may gain Christ and be found in him" (Phil 3:8).

---

6. Ignatius, *To the Trallians*, 4.
7. Ignatius, *To the Romans*, 6.

Everything allows for no exceptions. Not the prospect of dominion, nor that of popular acclaim; not a life of ease, nor indulgence; not long life, nor good health. In context, Ignatius urges his Roman brothers to refrain from attempting to circumvent his impending martyrdom. That is, on the basis of worldly considerations, and not in keeping with a willingness to suffer for Christ's sake.

Ignatius' dwelling on his coming martyrdom does not preclude his concern to minister as the occasion presents itself. As an example, "Do nothing without the bishop; keep your flesh as a temple of God; cherish union; shun divisions; be imitators of Jesus Christ, as He Himself also was of His Father."[8] His appeal to ecclesiastical authority concerns the apostolic tradition. It is in this regard that he urges his readers to *cherish union* and *shun divisions*.

So, also, they were to consider their bodies *as a temple of God*. Hence, free from any pollution. In this manner, emulating Jesus—who revealed the righteousness of his Father. Whether through life or death, reflecting a holy resolve.

"And why then have I delivered myself over to death, unto fire, unto sword, unto wild beasts?" Ignatius rhetorically inquires. "But near to the sword, near to God; in company with wild beasts, in company with God."[9] Suffering is not an end in itself, but only as it serves a worthwhile purpose.

In this connection, pain can be all consuming—so that nothing is to be gained. Or, on the other hand, it can serve God's redemptive purposes. It is in the latter regard that Ignatius can confidently affirm *near to the sword, near to God,* and *in company with wide beasts, in company with God.*

8. Ignatius, *To the Philadelphians*, 4.
9. Ignatius, *To the Smyraens*, 4.

Finally, "A Christian has no authority over himself, but gives his time to God. This is God's work, and yours also, when you shall complete it: for I trust in the Divine grace, that you are ready of an act of well-doing which is meet for God."[10] On the one hand, martyrdom constitutes a divine summons. On the other, one must determine whether he or she is a candidate.

Readiness is a critical factor. Consequently, one should not press on before it is time. Neither should one lag behind when the occasion presents itself. Qualifications aside, it is a relatively rare privilege accorded the martyr.

Thus primed, we turn our attention to the dramatic account of Polycarp's martyrdom. Irenaeus appreciatively recalls the venerable bishop:

> But Polycarp also was not only instructed by apostles, and conversed with many who had seen Christ, but was also, by apostles in Asia, appointed bishop of the Church in Smyrna, whom I also saw in my early youth, for he tarried a very long time, and when a very old man, gloriously and most nobly suffering martyrdom departed this life, having always taught the things which he had learned from the apostles, and which the Church has handed down, and down, and which alone are true.[11]

Smyrna, in turn, was located on the Aegean shoreline.

> (It) grew to be one of the most prosperous cities in Asia Minor. It was the natural port for the ancient trade route through the Hermus valley, and its im-

---

10. Ignatius, *To Polycarp*, 7.
11. Irenaeus, *Against Heresies*, III, 3, 4.

> mediate hinterland was very fertile. The city was a faithful ally of Rome long before Roman power became supreme in the eastern Mediterranean. Under the empire it was famous for its beauty and for the magnificence of its public buildings.[12]

Hence, it was a major center which solicited the bishop's devoted service.

It appears that the account of Polycarp's martyrdom does not date later than the middle of the second century, except for alleged interpolations—notoriously difficult to establish with any certainty. As for its purpose, succinctly expressed: "We write unto you, brothers, an account of what befell those that suffered martyrdom and especially the blessed Polycarp, who stayed the persecution, having as it were set his seal upon it by his martyrdom."[13]

"Now the glorious Polycarp at the first, when he heard it, so far from being dismayed was desirous of remaining in town; but the greater part persuaded him to withdraw" (5). So he withdrew to a farm not far distant from the city, where he stayed with a few companions. Here he spent his time in prayer, as was his custom.

When the search persisted, he moved on to another farm. There they overtook him. He conversed and persuaded them to allow him additional time for prayer. "They that heard were amazed, and many repented that they had come against such a venerable old man" (7).

Upon returning to the city, the bishop was met by the captain of police and his father, who attempted to persuade him to compromise his convictions. "What harm is there in

12. Bimson (ed.), *Baker Encyclopedia of Bible Places*, 287.

13. *The Martyrdom of Polycarp*, 1.

saying, 'Caesar is Lord,' and offering incense," they inquired, and thus "saving your-self?" (8). Although they persisted, he would not heed their counsel.

When he had entered the stadium, a voice enjoined him from heaven: "Be strong, Polycarp, and play the man" (9). No one saw the speaker, but *those of our people* who were present heard the voice. When his arrival was announced, a great tumult greeted him—ostensibly not unlike that which was directed against Paul's companions in Ephesus (cf. Acts 19:28–34).

The proconsul subsequently urged him: "Swear by the genius of Caesar; repent and say, 'Away with the atheists.'" This was a reference to the Christians, who refused to worship pagan deities.

Solemnly surveying the heathen crowded into the stadium, the bishop waved his hand in acknowledgment, and looking up toward heaven, petitioned: "Away with the atheists." When the magistrate continued to press him, he replied; "Fourscore and six years have I been His servant, and He has done me no wrong. How then can I blaspheme my King who saved me?"

Again failing to persuade Polycarp, the proconsul threatened: "I have beasts here and I will throw you to them, except you repent" (11).

"Call them," the bishop resolutely replied, "for the repentance from better to worse is a change not permitted to us; but is a noble thing to change from untowardness to righteousness." Then, with the prospect of being consumed by fire, he responded: "You threaten that fire which burns for a season and after a little while is quenched: for you are ignorant of the fire of the future judgment and eternal punishment, which is reserved for the ungodly."

Whereupon, the herald proclaimed three times: "Polycarp has confessed himself to be a Christian" (12). In response, the populace cried out for his execution.

When bound to a stake, *the noble man* prayed: "May I be received among those in Your presence this day, as a rich and acceptable sacrifice, as You have prepared and revealed it beforehand, and has accomplished it. You that are the faithful and true God" (14). To whom be glory *for the ages to come. Amen.*

When he had finished praying, the fire was lit. Then the flames seemed to form something resembling a vault, so that the body was not consumed. Instead, "we perceived such a fragrant smell, as if it were the wafted odor of frankincense or some other precious spice" (15).

At length, *the lawless men*—seeing that his body would not be consumed—ordered the executioner to stab him with a dagger. When this was done, there came forth a quantity of blood—so that the fire was extinguished. Then "all the multitude marveled that there should be so great a difference between the unbelievers and the elect" (16).

"So it befell the blessed Polycarp, who having with those from Philadelphia suffered martyrdom in Smyrna—twelve in all—is especially remembered more than the others by all men, so that he is talked of even by the heathen in every place" (19). Since "he who showed himself not only a notable teacher, but also a distinguished martyr, whose martyrdom all desire to imitate, seeing that it was after the pattern of the Gospel of Christ." So that in death he was able to extend his ministry, and sow what others would eventually reap. This was in accord with Tertullian's observation that *the blood of the martyrs is seed.*

The suffering of the martyr can be viewed as *travail*, in that it resembles a new birth. Where other efforts fail to achieve the desired results, it is necessary for one to put his or her life on the line. Consequently, it serves as a testimony to truth.

Qualifications aside, it would appear that the Christian martyr was inclined to embrace his calling with alacrity. In keeping with this thesis, Paul writes: "For me to live is Christ and to die is gain.... Yet what shall I choose? I do not know! I am torn between the two: I desire to depart and be with Christ, which is better by far; but it is more necessary for you that I remain in the body" (Phil 1:21–24). It is for the Almighty to make the call, so as to serve his redemptive purpose.

5

A Reasoned Faith

A YOUNG man was visibly taken back when I identified C. S. Lewis as a noted Christian apologist. He had appreciatively read the author over the years, quite enamored by his engaging literary style. Now he felt challenged to read him from a different perspective. "Who is going to harm you if you are eager to do good?" Peter rhetorically inquires:

> But even if you should suffer for what is right, you are blessed. Do not fear what they fear; do not be frightened. But in your hearts set apart Christ as Lord. Always be prepared to give an answer to everyone who asks you to give the reason for the hope that you have. But do this with gentleness and respect, keeping a clear conscience, so that those who speak maliciously against your good behavior in Christ may be ashamed of their slander. (1 Peter 3:13-16)

Such is the nature of Christian apologetics: *to give the reason for the hope that you have.* Not in a haughty or confrontational manner, but *with gentleness and respect*—in good conscience.

"During his years as an agnostic (otherwise identified as an atheist), Lewis wanted to know the answers to such questions as why God allows pain, why Christianity—out of all other religions—was held to be the true one, why and if miracles actually happen."[1] As a result, he quite naturally anticipated the questions others ask along these lines.

> After his conversion in 1931, Lewis, who seldom refused an invitation to speak or write about the Faith, found himself moving in very different circles. He preached to and argued with fellow dons, industrial workers, members of the Royal Air Force, and university students. (He reached the conclusion) that if you found it difficult to answer questions from men of different trades it was probably because "You haven't really thought it out; not to the end; not to 'the absolute ruddy end."[2]

The Problem of Pain is vintage Lewis. Herein he deftly reasons concerning suffering from a Christian perspective. As for the dilemma, consider the case of a Jewish friend, who could not bring himself to exercise faith in God—given the tragic event of the Holocaust. He confided in me that his wife and children were religious, and he wished he could bring himself to share their confidence. However, the problem of pain resolutely stood in the way.

Lewis admits at the outset that he had forsaken the faith in which he was raised. If asked why he did not believe in God, he would point out the vast extent of the universe, the uncertainty of whether life exists elsewhere, and the recent arrival of mankind on the scene. Upon further reflection, "The creatures cause pain by being born, and live by inflicting pain, and in pain they mostly die."[3]

---

1. Lewis, (Hooper, ed.), *God in the Dock*, 8.
2. Ibid.
3. Lewis, *The Problem of Pain*, 14.

Moreover, this is coupled in man with reason, to allow humans to anticipate pain and their eventual demise. "Their history is largely a record of crime, war, disease, and terror, with just sufficient happiness interposed to give them, while it lasts, an agonized apprehension of losing it, and, when it is lost, the poignant misery of remembering."

Even so, there was one question that Lewis never dreamed of raising: "If the universe is so bad, or even half so bad, how on earth did human beings ever come to attribute it to the activity of a wise and good Creator?" This would seem to be an extremely unlikely scenario. Unless, that is, there were some other compelling line of evidence to account for the phenomenon.

As a matter of record, he observes that there are three elements found in all *developed religion*, and with regard to Christianity a fourth. Initially, there is the *numinous* experience. Suppose, one were told that there was a tiger in the next room. He or she would rightly conclude that life was at risk.

If, however, we were told that there was a ghost present, the fear accompanying it would be of a different sort. Namely, since it is an unnatural creature, making one uncertain as how to proceed.

Then, should a person be alerted to a mighty spirit in the room, this would be even less like a simple fear of danger but that of profound inadequacy. To which we attach the term *awe*, as in the refrain: "Our God is an awesome God." Either this constitutes a mere twist of the human mind, corresponding to nothing objective and serving no legitimate purpose; or it is an awareness of the supernatural. In addition, we are encouraged to embrace the simpler of the two scenarios, what is described in philosophic jargon as *Occam's razor*.

Secondly, humans acknowledge some sort of morality, as expressed in terms of what we ought or ought not to do. Morality, like the experience of numinous, requires that we go beyond what can be observed to account for it in some other fashion. What might be described as *sufficient cause*.

Then, too, there is the sense that we violate the code of morality. Not only in given specifics, but as a regretful matter of course. This leaves us with the possibility that this is either an inexplicable illusion or else reflecting the actual state of our existence. Again, we do well to opt for the more likely alternative.

Thirdly, we discover that in some religions the experience of numinous and morality are associated. The object of our numinous experience thus assumes the role of our moral guardian. Consequently, to violate the moral code is to put ourselves in serious jeopardy. Lewis singles out the Jewish tradition as a prime example of this phenomenon. In particular, the Jews perceived themselves to be a chosen people—meant to reveal the righteous ways of the Almighty. In more graphic terms, they were to serve as a light to the Gentiles.

Finally,

> There was a man born among these Jews who claimed to be, or to be the son of, or to be "one with" the Something which is at once the awful haunter of nature and the giver of the moral law. The claim is so shocking—a paradox, and even a horror, which we may easily be lulled into taking too lightly—that only two views of this man are possible.[4]

---

4. Ibid., 23.

Either he was a raving lunatic of an unusually abominable type, or he was expressly what he claimed to be. It comes as no surprise that Lewis opts for the latter alternative, and thus the course is set for subsequent reflection.

The apologist wastes no time in focusing his attention on the problem associated with divine omnipotence. In brief, if God were good, he would not want to inflict pain on his creatures, and if he were omnipotent, he could refrain from doing so. Since humans suffer, either God is not good, all powerful, or both. Or, another option, he simply does not exist.

As an aside, my philosophy professor at the university opted for a finite god as a way out of the dilemma. Consequently, he proposed that God was doing his best, and earnestly solicited our cooperation. Lewis refuses this tempting way out.

Initially, he points out that omnipotence conveys the notion of being able to do anything intrinsically possible. For instance, God cannot make a round square—since this is a contradiction in terms. Of greater import, the Almighty will not violate his righteous disposition, because this too would amount to an inherent contradiction.

Along a related line, our use of the term *impossible* implies the notion of *unless*. Thus it is impossible to see the street from where I am sitting, *unless* I walk to the window. This, in turn, reminds us of the conditional character that qualifies what one can or cannot do.

So it is that God cannot create both creatures with and without freedom to choose. If the former, the stakes go up immeasurably, whether for good or evil. If the latter, God opts for a lesser being—presumably ill-suited to be cast in the divine image.

Also, this requires a neutral setting. It is one where miracles may occur, but not with such frequency that they set aside the predictable order of things. In this connection, it should be noted the frequency of miracles increases at critical junctures in salvation history—such as with the exodus, struggle of the Hebrew prophets with Baalism, and in the time of Jesus and the apostles. They may occur more frequently than we realize, in other connections, since we may be conditioned not to recognize them.

Whereupon, Lewis shifts his focus to divine goodness. On the one hand, his perception of what is good assuredly transcends our own. On the other hand, there must be some correlation between the two, if morality is to make any sense. Furthermore, this correlation may be considerably improved by cultivating God's righteous ways.

The apologist recalls that when he matriculated to the university, he was as nearly without a moral consciousness as a young person might be. Fortunately, he fell in with students whose moral sensitivity was more advanced than his own, and from whom he greatly benefitted. This incited him to reflect more at length on the character of God's compassion for his human creatures.

There is, for instance, the compelling interest an artisan has for his artifact. "O house of Israel, can I not do with you as this potter does?" the Lord inquires. "Like clay in the hand of the potter, so are you in my hand" (Jer 18:6).

Still more revealing is the concern expressed regarding the animals we tend. Along this line, "The Lord is my shepherd, I shall not want. He makes me lie down in green pastures, he leads me beside quiet waters, he restores my soul" (Ps 23:1–3). He guides me in the paths of righteousness, and through the menacing ravines. "Surely goodness and love (like two guard dogs) will follow me all the days of my life, and I will dwell in the house of the Lord forever."

A nobler analogy consists of God's love for his offspring. As currently expressed, it amounts to *hard love*. Consequently, Lewis pointedly observes: since God loves us, he means to make us lovable. In this regard, Jesus enjoined his disciples to pray: "Our Father in heaven, hallowed be your name, your kingdom come, your will be done on earth as it is in heaven" (Matt 6:9).

"The problem of reconciling human suffering with the existence of a God who loves," Lewis abruptly concludes, "is only insoluble so long as we attach a trivial meaning to the word 'love,' and look on things as if man were the center of them."[5] Man is not the center. God does not exist for the sake of his creature, but the reverse. It goes without saying that what is good for God is best for humans.

Would that man were as readily disposed. The Christian tradition insists that man has abused his privileges, resulting in alienation and anguish. Lewis supposes that this is a harder sell today than in former times. This brings to mind Francis Schaeffer's observation some years ago that he felt compelled to spend eighty percent of his energies in pre-evangelism. As otherwise expressed, one needs to realize that he or she is lost before appreciating the need to be saved.

In this regard, Lewis reasons that the worst thing we could have done is to turn our backs on the Almighty. If we are content to leave him alone, why isn't he willing to leave us alone? It is easy enough for him to do good.

5. Ibid., 48.

How are we to escape this *fool's illusion*? First, by refusing to compare ourselves with others. By assuming that we are better than someone else; if not in every regard, then in some. As in the instance of a person who boasted that while he had done much that was wrong, he did not try to conceal his faults—as others with whom he was unfortunately acquainted.

Second, beware that in focusing on corporate guilt we overlook those *humdrum* faults of our own, which compound the problem. It is all too easy to put the blame on society, in general terms or concerning some specific.

Third, do not suppose that time is a panacea for all our faults. When, in fact, time tends to confirm us in the way we have chosen. In another context, Lewis reasons that only God knows when time will no longer serve a constructive purpose.

Fourth, guard against the impression that there is safety in numbers. "Enter through the narrow gate," Jesus aptly admonished. "For wide is the gate and broad is the road that leads to destruction, and many enter through it. But small is the gate and narrow the road that leads to life, and only a few find it" (Matt 7:13–14).

Fifth, do not suppose that our society is somehow immune from the perversity that characterized former ages. While cultures differ from one another, none are so pristine as to escape God's scathing rebuke. Moreover, the apologist elsewhere encourages us to read one old book for each new one, since we are more likely to recognize the short-comings of the past than the present. In this manner, we may be alerted to our own degradation.

Sixth, do not reduce the moral code to being kind one to the other. Even a virtue like pity, if not controlled by love and justice, leads through anger to cruelty. As a result, most atrocities are stimulated by accounts of the enemy's savagery, and concern for the oppressed classes in and of itself can lead to the brutalities of a reign of terror.

Seventh, recognize that the road to the promised land runs past Sinai. In other words, while our response to the Almighty ought not to be reduced to a moral code, neither should we dismiss moral considerations. According to conventional wisdom, we learn in order that we might do.

Eighth, "When tempted, no one should say, 'God is tempting me'" (Jas 1:13). Many would have us shift the responsibility of our behavior from our own shoulders to some inherent necessity, thus indirectly to the Sovereign Lord.

Lewis concludes this chapter with reference to the doctrine of total depravity. Worthy of note, *total depravity* does not mean that persons are necessarily as bad as they could be, but our sinful inclination is pervasive. In this regard, evil plagues our reason, emotions, and volition.

How did this situation come about? In brief, Lewis suggests that it is good gone wrong. Our present condition, consequently, is explained by the fact that we are members of a spoiled species. Not that we are personally at fault for this defection, but that we compound it by our willful disobedience. As noted in another context, there is more than enough blame to go around.

The apologist reasons that suffering is inherent in a world where humans interact. Moreover,

> When souls become wicked they will certainly use this possibility to hurt one another; and this, perhaps, accounts for four-fifths of the sufferings of men. It is men, not God, who have produced racks, whips, prisons, slavery, guns, bayonets, and bombs; it is by human avarice or human stupidity, not by the churlishness of nature, that we have poverty and overwork.[6]

As for the rest, pain can serve a constructive purpose—in that it may incite human contrition. Humans are disinclined to amend their ways so long as things go well. As graphically expressed by Lewis, *God whispers to us in our pleasures, speaks to our conscience, but shouts in our pain.* As previously noted, he allows that God is more inclined to employ *carrots* (incentives) than *clubs* (coercion). In addition, pain arises from the conditions of our situation, rather than being imposed upon us.

Lewis subsequently sets forth six propositions, meant to firm up his contention. First, there is a paradox concerning suffering from a Christian perspective. "Blessed are those who are persecuted because of righteousness," Jesus assured his disciples, "for theirs is the kingdom of heaven" (Matt 5:10). As Lewis points out, this does not mean that pain is good in itself, but that it can serve a constructive purpose.

Second, since suffering is involved in human redemption, we ought not to suppose that it will cease until that redemption is complete. "A Christian cannot, therefore, believe any of those who promise that if only some reforms in our economic, political, or hygiene systems were made, a heaven on earth would follow."[7]

6. Ibid., 89.
7. Ibid., 114.

Third, there is no precise correlation between a Christian orientation and any of the alternative political systems. The apologist thus implies that political structures are approximate means, not to be confused with the kingdom of God.

Fourth, the settled security and happiness we desire remains future—although we enjoy an earnest of it in the present. Or, as graphically expressed by Lewis, while our Father refreshes us on the journey with some pleasant inns, he encourages us not to mistake them for home.

Sixth, suffering is deprived of its malicious effect when employed by God for a constructive purpose. Lewis identifies the *complex good* in this context, as that which God expresses towards humans in their fallen estate.

The apologist touches on three related issues in conclusion: hell and heaven, along with the pain experienced by animals. Disregarding his order, animal pain first invites our consideration. Lewis discounts the idea that it was essentially due to human defection, although this could be a contributing factor. Conversely, he allows that it could be caused by satanic corruption. In any case, it ought not to prejudice our understanding of the human dilemma.

As for commentary, there is a human world quite distinct from all else. The same could presumably be said of the cat or dog world. However, these overlap the human world—especially when it comes to domesticated animals. Lewis speculates at some length whether these might enjoy a future existence, given their peculiar relationship to man. However, the bottom line is that we simply do not know.

Backtracking, we pick up on the notion of *hell*. The apologist allows that this is one of the chief grounds on which Christianity is impugned as being barbarous, and the goodness of God questioned. As such, it is said to be *a detestable doctrine*.

It is in the above context that the apologist sets out to answer five objections. Initially, certain persons protest any form of retributive justice. In response, Lewis points out that retribution takes the form of a reality check. It serves in this capacity to dissuade persons from the delusion that they have beaten the system, and got the better of God and one's fellow man.

The demand that God should forgive such a person reveals a confusion between condoning and forgiving. "To condone an evil is simply to ignore it, to treat it as if it were good. But forgiveness needs to be accepted as well as offered if it is to be complete: and a man who admits no guilt can accept no forgiveness."[8]

Another objection turns on the apparent disproportion between eternal damnation and transitory sin. This arises from thinking of eternity as simply an extension of time, which Lewis thinks is an unlikely case. In any case, the ambiguity at this point cautions us not to base our criticism on the unknown.

There also is concern expressed regarding the frightful intensity of the punishment, portrayed as unrelenting flames. Lewis cautions us in this regard not to confuse reality with its imagery. To illustrate his thesis, the thing that impressed me most concerning the Valley of Hinnom—which served as a smoldering rubbish dump in Jesus' time, was it embraced that which was no longer usable for the purpose for which it was intended.

Fourth, it is said that no charitable person could be content in heaven while knowing that another suffered in hell.

8. Ibid., 122.

The apologist points out that this objection evolves from the idea that heaven and hell constitute two parallel accommodations, a problematic conclusion at best. In proverbial terms, the more we know about such things the more we realize we do not know.

Fifth, it is alleged that the loss of even one soul amounts to a failure of divine omnipotence. "What you call defeat, I call a miracle," Lewis unabashedly counters: "for to make things which are not itself, and thus to become, in a sense, capable of being resisted by its own handiwork, is the most astonishing and unimaginable of all the feats we attribute to the Deity."[9]

As for *heaven*, it offers nothing that a mercenary soul would desire. Here diverse persons bring to the worship of God their several spiritual legacies. All this is carefully orchestrated to bring glory to the Almighty.

Thus persons also will be enabled to share with and receive from others—as a means of blessing, and resulting in blessing. In incomparable fashion, as the former limitations have been done away with. In inconceivable ways, since fellowship invites creative expression.

All things considered, it would seem that Lewis is of the opinion that we are more pulled by the future than driven by the past. In this connection, "Everyone who has this hope in him purifies himself, just as he (God) is pure" (1 John 3:3). Whereupon, seizing on every opportunity, pleasure and pain alike, press on with confidence in the divine promises. Be assured that God wills it!

---

9. Ibid., 127.

6

Highlights

Not uncommonly when returning from a journey, I reflect on some of its more memorable events. In like manner, I thought back over some of the salient points in the preceding discussion—concerning pain as a means of grace. These will serve not only to sharpen the focus, but prime the reader for additional deliberation.

The stage was set by a story regarding a young couple who were informed that the child they were enthusiastically expecting would be severely handicapped. "The wife subsequently gave birth. Time passed, and the parents came to appreciatively refer to it as their *love child*."

This graphically illustrates at the outset that the human capacity for pleasure is comparable to that for pain. If more of the one, then seemingly more of the other. So one would conclude that the stakes go up concerning humans, as created in the divine image.

Otherwise, this would appear a contradiction of terms. In this regard, divine omnipotence connotes the ability to do all things that are not mutually exclusive. Such as create a being that has and at the same time does not have certain capacities.

Furthermore, it is axiomatic in Hebrew thought that life is good. Provided, that is, that it is lived according to God's benevolent design. Otherwise, we can expect things to go from bad to worse.

"Now the Lord God had planted a garden in the east, in Eden, and there he put the man he had formed. And the Lord God made all kinds of trees grow out of the ground—trees that were pleasing to the eye and good for food" (Gen 2:9). Whereupon, the Lord God informed man: "You are free to eat from any tree in the garden, but you must not eat from the tree of the knowledge of good and evil, for when you eat of it you will surely die."

Man opted to violate the prohibition, much as a willful child who rejects the loving constraint of its parent. Then, having done so, it falls prey to every sort of misadventure. The bad news was that man was cast out of the garden paradise, and prohibited from returning. The good news was that God had not utterly forsaken him. Henceforth, he would experience what Lewis aptly describes as *complex good*, resulting from God's continued concern expressed in a fallen condition.

While it does not say that travail was altogether without pain, it was heightened as a result of the fall. Thus, as previously noted, the original ideal of *to love and to cherish* was usurped by desire and domination.

Turning to Adam, God declares: "Cursed is the ground because of you; through painful toil you will eat of it all the days of your life." Thus, while industry is portrayed as normal and fulfilling, it here becomes burdensome and unrewarding. In particular, nature appears as uncooperative.

All things considered, *paradise lost* thus reflects a scenario where the prospect of pleasure is minimized, while that of pain enhanced. In a manner of speaking, the parameters have been altered for the worse. So things will remain, until the time of restoration. Accordingly, we are reminded that while God blesses us in transit, this world is not our final destination.

Not to be overlooked, there is the adversary—represented by the serpent. Although the creature might convey a variety of things from antiquity; the notion of deception seems paramount here. This concept persists in Arab culture with an irregular motion of the hand, as over against someone who is straightforward.

Even so, why do the godly suffer sometimes disproportionately to the rest? Within the constraints of our limited understanding, the Job narrative attempts a reply. While the patriarch was not without fault, he was exemplary. Satan proposes that this was because he hoped to get special consideration. God allows that he be tested.

Initially, the test concerns his family circle and vast possessions. He remains firm. The test then extends to his person. Again, he remains firm. This is eminently expressed by his observation, "The Lord gave and the Lord has taken away; may the name of the Lord be praised" (1:21).

His *friends* compound the problem by their simplistic and insensitive suggestions. The patriarch deserved better. As a result, God informed Eliphaz, "I am angry with you and your friends, because you have not spoken of me what is right, as my servant Job has" (42:7). God has the final word.

What are we to learn from all this? First, that God is deserving of our unqualified approval. "Ascribe to the Lord the glory due his name," the psalmist enjoins; "worship the Lord in the splendor of his holiness" (29:1). Accordingly, without exception, and without restraint.

Second, embrace divine omnipotence in the context of all things working together for good for those who love him and are called according to his purpose. Consequently, what some would consider a repudiation of God's sovereignty, C. S. Lewis views as a miracle of his grace.

Finally, recognize that God's ways are often mysterious. Sometimes less so when we have had an opportunity to reflect back on them. In all probability, as a testimony to his creativeness. Consequently, opting for the way of the righteous, as opposed to that of the wicked: the Job narrative serves us well in this regard.

There is a natural transition between the experience of Job and that of Jesus' passion. As for commentary, Ben Witherington III allows:

> I should repeat from the outset that I do not think any one term or title fully captures the truth about the historical Jesus.... But if we ask what heuristic category comes closest to explaining the most about who Jesus thought he was and what he said and did, what comes closest to explaining why early Christological thinking about Jesus developed as it did, then we must come to grips with sages and Wisdom.[1]

It comes as no surprise that commentators dwell at length on the physical aspects of Jesus' suffering. The cross loomed large on the horizon as his public ministry progressed. "And being in anguish, he prayed more earnestly,

---

1. Witherington III, *The Jesus Quest*, 185.

and his sweat was like drops of blood falling to the ground" (Luke 22:44). If an instance of hematridrosis, as the physician Alexander Metherell supposes, a severe anxiety causes the release of chemicals that break down the capillaries in the sweat glands.

This, in turn, would have elevated Jesus' suffering when flogged. He was in a greatly weakened condition when facing the ordeal of crucifixion. Characteristically an extended death by asphyxiation, Jesus succumbed more quickly.

There was in addition the emotional distress caused by rejection, deprivation, antagonism, and defection. The combination of which made his lot the more difficult to bear, as the course of his ministry unfolded.

"The real meaning of the cross of the Lord is the pain of God," Kazoh Kitamori succinctly concludes. "To follow the Lord of the cross is to serve the pain of God."[2] In context, he reasons that the experience of Jesus internalized pain for the Almighty. This would seem eminently plausible.

Then, too, Christian discipleship departs by way of the cross. As previously noted, the Christian is not allowed to determine the conditions under which he will suffer: whether alone or with others, whether ridiculed or applauded, whether recalled as a sinner or a saint. "So it is that the long shadow of the cross extends throughout succeeding generations."

We subsequently explored how this impacted on the lot of the martyrs. First Stephen, then Ignatius, and finally Polycarp. Stephen is described as a person *full of God's grace and power*. Opposition arose from among the Hellenistic Jews, but *they could not stand up against the wisdom of the Spirit by whom he spoke*.

2. Kitamori, *Theology of the Pain of God*, 50.

He was seized and brought before the Sanhedrin. Certain charged him with departing from the sacred tradition. He responded by alluding to the intransigence of those up to the present by resisting the Holy Spirit. Whereupon, he gazed upward intently, declaring that he saw heaven open and *the Son of Man standing at the right hand of God*. At this, they covered their ears, and shouting at the top of their voices, dragged him out of the city and began to stone him. In turn, he prayed on their behalf. Stephen is remembered as the first of the Christian martyrs.

Others would follow over the course of time. In particular, we turned our attention to Ignatius. He was a disciple of John, who governed the church at Antioch. This congregation was founded by some who had fled the persecution following Stephen's demise. It would eventually boast an impressive group of prophets and teachers. It was also from here that Paul and Barnabas set out on their first missionary journey.

"Ignatius composed seven extant epistles while in transit from Antioch to Rome, where he would suffer martyrdom." Herein, he reflects on his coming demise. As a result, we are able to piece together the prospect of suffering from the martyr's perspective. While not all would be called upon to embrace martyrdom, all are admonished to entertain the possibility.

"And why then have I delivered myself over to death, unto fire, unto sword, unto wild beasts?" Ignatius rhetorically inquires. "But near to the sword, near to God; in company with wild beasts, in company with God." In this regard, "It is good for me to die for Jesus Christ rather than to reign over the farthest bounds of the earth."

His focus on the coming martyrdom did not exclude his continuing concern for the welfare of the churches. He urges prayer on their behalf, and that they strive for unity. This, in turn, was in keeping with the apostolic tradition.

Polycarp serves as a final example. When notified that the authorities were in search of him, he purposed to stand fast. When persuaded to withdraw, he spent his time in prayer. When apprehended, he went peacefully. When enjoined to deny Christ, he adamantly refused.

Upon being bound to a stake, he prayed: "May I be received among those in Your presence this day, as a rich and acceptable sacrifice, as You have prepared and revealed it beforehand, and have accomplished it, You that are the faithful and true God." To whom be glory *for the ages to come. Amen.*

Consequently, it is recalled that "he showed himself not only a notable teacher, but also a distinguished martyr, whose martyrdom all desire to imitate, seeing that it was after the pattern of the Gospel of Christ." So that with his death he was able to greatly extend his fervent ministry.

All things considered, the Christian martyr seems to have characteristically entertained his suffering with alacrity. This was in keeping with the conviction that it served as the ultimate expression of his or her sanctification, served in the larger purpose of God's redemptive design, and as sustained by God's lavish grace. "Therefore we conquer in dying," Tertullian confidently concludes, "we go forth victorious at the very time we are subdued."[3]

While the martyr naturally comes to mind concerning suffering for the cause of the gospel, this serves simply as the tip of the proverbial iceberg. Most are called upon to embrace

3. Tertullian, *The Apology*, L.

pain in the process of living a full and godly life. C. S. Lewis qualifies as a prime example.

He came to the task of a Christian apologist by way of his own earlier uncertainties. This allowed him to anticipate the questions others would be asking, and to formulate a reasonable response. This comprised more than an intellectual exercise for him, as it was a matter of uttermost importance.

Lewis approached the problem of pain via religious intuition. In particular, he points out that there are three elements found in developed religion, to which Christianity adds a fourth. There is the experience of numinous—which incites awe, morality, and the combination of the two. Then, with the Christian faith, there is the incarnation.

Having set the course, the apologist discusses divine omnipotence, and then goodness. Each requires clarification: the former so as to disallow anything that is inherently contradictory, and the latter as what translates into *hard love*—or as he observes, because God loves us he seeks to make us lovable.

Lewis takes something of a pastoral approach at this juncture, encouraging his readers not to compare themselves with others, focus on corporate guilt so as to overlook our own, or to suppose that time is a panacea for all our faults. Likewise, to guard against the impression that there is safety in numbers, the supposition that our society is somehow immune from the perversity expressed in former ages, the temptation to reduce morality to kindness, and the inclination to blame God for our duplicity.

He subsequently touches on several related topics: human pain, hell, animal pain, and heaven. For instance, the apologist concludes that hell accommodates those who will accept nothing better from a compassionate deity. In this regard, he cautions us not to confuse reality with the imagery.

It bears repeating, "To condone an evil is simply to ignore it, to treat it as if it were good. But forgiveness needs to be accepted as well as offered if it is to be complete: and a man who admits no guilt can accept no forgiveness."

Since this journey began with a story—concerning the *love child*, it seems proper to conclude with one. Sarah was a happy person, and a joy to be around. Consequently, her uninhibited laughter recalls pleasant moments. It was subsequently brought to my attention that she had encountered trying difficulties and discouragements in the course of her life. However, instead of being disheartened by this, her Christian faith caused her to rise to the occasion. As a result, she bore witness to the notion of *pain as a means of grace.*

Bibliography

Anderson, Francis. *Job*. Downers Grove: InterVarsity, n.d.

Bimson, John (ed.). *Baker Encyclopedia of Biblical Resources*. Grand Rapids: Baker, 1995.

Bruce, F. D. *The Gospel of John*, Grand Rapids: Eerdmans, 1983.

Eckstein, Yechiel. *How Firm a Foundation*. Brewster: Paraclete, 1997.

Hagner, Donald. *Matthew 14–28*. Dallas: Word, 1995.

Ignatius. *To the Ephesians*.

———. *To the Philadelphians*.

———. *To Polycarp*.

———. *To the Romans*.

———. *To the Smyraens*.

———. *To the Trallians*.

Inch, Morris. *Exhortations of Jesus According to Matthew* and *Up From the Depths*. Lanham: University Press of America, 1997.

———. *My Servant Job*. Grand Rapids: Baker, 1979.

———. *Scripture As Story*. Lanham: University Press of America. 2000.

Irenaeus. *Against Heresies*.

Kitamori, Kazoh. *Theology of the Pain of God*. Richmond: John Knox, 1965.

Lane, William. *The Gospel of Mark*. Grand Rapids: Eerdmans, 1974.

Lewis, C. S. *God in the Dock,* edited by Walter Hooper. Grand Rapids: Eerdmans, 1970.

———. *The Problem of Pain*. New York: Macmillan, 1962.

The Martyrdom of Ignatius.

The Martyrdom of Polycarp.

Milton, John. *Paradise Lost*.

Steinberg, Milton. *Basic Judaism*. New York: Harcourt, Brace & World, 1947.

Strobel, Lee. *The Case For Christ*. Grand Rapids: Zondervan, 1998.
Tertullian. *The Apology*.
Wenham, Gordon. *Genesis 1-15*. Dallas: Word, 1987.
Williams, David. *Acts*. Peabody: Hendrickson, 1993.
Witherington, Ben III. *The Jesus Quest*. InterVarsity. 1997.

www.ingramcontent.com/pod-product-compliance
Lightning Source LLC
Chambersburg PA
CBHW070059100426
42743CB00012B/2591